No Sugar, No Problem

The Sugar-Free Dieter's Weight Loss Survival Guide

J.C. Collins

**Limits of Liability, Disclaimer of Warranties & Terms of
Use**
This book is a general educational health-related information
product. As an express condition to reading this book, you
understand and agree to following terms. The information and
advice contained in this book are not intended as a substitute for
consulting with a healthcare professional.

The publisher and authors are not responsible for any adverse
effects or consequences resulting from the use of any of the
suggestions, or procedures discussed in this book. While all
attempts have been made to verify information provided in this
book, the author and publisher assume no responsibility for
errors, omissions, or contrary interpretation of the subject
matter herein. All matters pertaining to your physical health
should be supervised by a health care professional

ISBN-10: 1500429899
ISBN-13: 978-1500429898

DEDICATION

This book is dedicated to those in search of an effective way to lose weight and eliminate belly fat through The Sugar-Free Diet.

CONTENTS

INTRODUCTION

This book contains proven steps and strategies on how to effectively lose weight and eliminate belly fat through The Sugar-Free Diet.

In the first chapter, you will learn the reasons why sugar can contribute to weight gain. Knowing the concept first will help you understand the whole process. In the second chapter, sugar-free diet will be introduced. In the third chapter, you will learn the different benefits you will gain once you start the sugar-free diet.

In the fourth chapter, you will learn certain rules of the sugar-free diet. In the fifth chapter, you will know the specific types of food you need to eat. Food restrictions are also provided in this chapter. In the sixth and last chapter, you will learn about other things you can do to maximize your weight loss.

CHAPTER 1 – TOP REASONS WHY SUGAR INTAKE RESULTS TO WEIGHT GAIN

Sugar intake does not only pertain to a spoonful of sugar you add into your coffee, juice, and desserts. Almost all of the processed foods available in the market, from drinks to meat, consist of sugar. Based on recent studies, the average sugar consumption of an American per week is more than one pound.

Sugar must not be taken for granted, as it can cause adverse effects to your body. Many people may not be totally aware that sugar can contribute to an increasing weight. Here are the top reasons why sugar can add to your waistline.

Insulin Resistance Caused by Fructose

- Insulin is a hormone that functions in controlling the body's metabolism and energy utilization. This hormone is produced by the pancreas and flows in the blood. It will be transported to different cells in the body. Insulin gives off signals, which indicate the cells to transport and convert glucose into energy.

- When your sugar intake is high, the glucose in your blood increases. Too much glucose in the blood may be detrimental to one's health, so the insulin will instruct the cells to take glucose away from the bloodstream. When insulin fails to work properly, glucose may become a toxic in the body. A similar case would happen if there is insufficient supply of insulin.

- Another function of the insulin is to send indicators to fat cells. The indicators will tell the fat cells to take fats away from the blood and stock them. Also, the fat cells are prohibited to burn fats. When your insulin level is high, the more fats will be stored in the fat cells.

- The main reason for having an insulin resistance and high insulin level is overindulgence in fructose. If this is the case, the brain will unconsciously send signals, indicating that you are hungry even if the body does not need food.

Leptin Resistance Caused by Fructose

- Leptin is a kind of hormone that is produced by fat cells. As the size of a fat cell increases, the quantity of leptin also increases. Once the brain sensed that there is an enough supply of leptin, it will order the body to refrain from eating foods. This is because you have already enough supply of fats, which will be converted to energy. If the body can throw signals for you to stop eating, then it may prevent you from being overweight. However, if the body becomes resistant to leptin, then you will feel hungry from time to time. In this way, you will end up eating more foods and burning less fat.

- The leptin-induced hunger is not easy to overcome. This is why many people find it difficult to lose weight. When your sugar intake is high, your body is at a greater risk of being leptin resistant.

Sugar is Incapable of Stimulating Satiety

Even if you fill your stomach with sugar-loaded foods, you will still feel hungry since sugar cannot induce satiety unlike any other food does. There is a hormone called ghrelin, which is also known as the hunger hormone. A study claimed that sugar does not have the ability to reduce the amount of ghrelin in the body. As a result, your brain is incapable of controlling your food intake.

Sugar has an Addictive Property

Sugar can stimulate dopamine and opiate activities in your brain center. These activities are also induced by certain drugs like cocaine. A research study found out that sugar has an addictive property, which is similar to illegal drugs. Researchers used rats as their model. They concluded that sugar can cause behavioral and neurochemical transformations, which bear a resemblance to the results of drug abuse.

Sugar intake gives happiness to many people. The release of opiates and dopamines take place in the nucleus accumbens, which is the same area where cocaine and nicotine are being stimulated. People who are suffering from sugar addiction are the ones who still overindulge in sweets despite of knowing the fact that it can disrupt their health.

Since many people are fond of eating sweets, they gain weight exponentially. If you don't want to become obese, read the next chapter to discover the most effective diet for curbing your sugar intake.

CHAPTER 2 – LOSING WEIGHT THROUGH SUGAR-FREE DIET

A person addicted to sugar may find it difficult to resist the temptation. Motivation is what you need to overcome your sugar cravings. Aside from losing weight, there are a lot of reasons why you should start a sugar-free diet. The short-term and long-term consequences of excessive sugar intake may cause adverse effects on our health.

Sugar can directly increase your weight

- When your sugar consumption is high, the blood sugar level will be elevated. If you are trying to lose weight, a high blood sugar level will not be advantageous on your part.

- The main requirement of the body to activate its fat burning system is a stable blood sugar level. Therefore, starting a sugar-free diet is the best option to do. If you want to lose weight, then sugar must be eliminated from your diet.

Sugar does not have any nutritional value

- Aside from giving you a sweet taste, sugar does not contribute any nutritional value to the body. Literally, sugar gives nothing to your body. When you eat sugar, you are actually overwhelming yourself with empty calories, which are difficult to metabolize.

- When your body does not completely metabolize carbohydrates, it may lead to the development of toxic metabolites – pyruvic acid and nonstandard sugar.

- Nonstandard sugars are comprised of 5-carbon molecules. Pyruvic acid goes into the nervous system while the nonstandard sugars accumulate in the erythrocytes.

- The cell respiration may be interrupted by these toxic metabolites. As a result, the cells will have an insufficient supply of oxygen, which may inhibit them to function normally. In some cases, cells may die if there is no oxygen at all. This means that sugar can kill our cells.

Sugar can disrupt the normal activities of your hormones

- Sugar is considered to be a strong hormone disruptor. When the hormones do not perform their function, your body will be disabled in maintaining system equilibrium.

- If leptin, insulin and ghrelin are disrupted, your body will be at a greater risk of increasing weight.

J.C. Collins

CHAPTER 3 – BENEFITS OF THE SUGAR-FREE DIET

It is not easy to eliminate your sugar intake, so you need to have a strong will power in order to curb sugar cravings completely. You may be encouraged to have a sugar-free diet once you learn about the several health benefits you can gain from it.

Here is a List of the Sugar-Free Diet Benefits:

You will be more resistant to various diseases.

- The body uses up its accumulated nutrients to metabolize sugar. If your sugar intake is high, the more nutrients will be consumed for sugar metabolism. Thus, nutrient deficiencies are caused by high sugar intake.

- Sugar can also affect your immune system. It interrupts in the production of growth hormones by increasing the insulin level. White blood cells

9

are utilized for cleaning up the waste brought by sugar. In this case, sugar inhibits the white blood cells to do its main function, which is to fight against the bacteria and diseases.

- It may also cause an inflammation throughout the body. An inflammation can lead to dermatitis, indigestion, hyperactivity and depression. The digestive system may also be affected. It may not absorb the nutrients properly if your sugar intake is high.

You can easily manage your hunger and cravings.

- In sugar metabolism, the body utilizes its stored nutrients – Vitamin B, potassium and chromium. As you consume sweets, the supply of nutrients decreases. Therefore, sugar can make a person unhealthy. Usually, sugar-loaded foods are less in nutrients. If you eat more sweets, then you are not satisfying the body's nutrient requirements.

- The body needs water, fat and protein to work properly. As long as you don't meet the nutrient requirements, you may feel hungry once in a while. Overindulging in foods usually happens when you eat more sugar than any other essential nutrient.

- If you follow a sugar-free diet, then you can prevent yourself from overindulging. As a result, your weight will be reduced. You should know what the right amount of food is and when is the right time to eat.

You can boost your energy and feel less tired.

When you consume sugar, the production of tryptophan is stimulated. Tryptophan will be transformed into serotonin, a sleeping hormone. If you are on a sugar-free diet, you usually eat whole and unrefined ingredients. These ingredients are full of antioxidants, fiber, protein, vitamins and water that bring fuel for the body and brain.

Your mental precision will be improved.

- A study shows that memory loss and incapability to focus are associated with sugar. You are more likely to feel nervous and think negatively. As sugar creates inflammation in the body, the chemistry of the brain is being affected.

Sugar-free diet can make you look good.

- The body needs vitamins and minerals to have bright eyes, smooth and silky skin, and healthy hair. Sugar is capable of getting nutrients away from your body. Therefore, consuming sugar can lead to loss of nutrients.

- Glycation is a process where sugar sticks with protein, leading to advanced glycation end products (AGE). A research proved that AGEs can cause loose skin and wrinkles.

You can easily control and sustain your weight.

- Eliminating sugar from your diet can lead to weight loss. The body needs fat, but excess fats should not be maintained. Usually, excess sugar is converted into fat cells.

You are at a lower risk of acquiring dental disorders.

- Sugar stimulates the proliferation of bacteria that cause teeth cavities. Although brushing your teeth can eradicate bacteria, it is not enough to remove tartars that build up on your teeth. This may lead to oral health disorders. A good solution for this problem is to use sugar substitutes such as Xylitol instead of consuming sugar. Xylitol may bring calories, but it will not cause cavities.

You can avoid allergens.

- Corn derivatives are used as additives in most processed foods, baked goods and pastries. Usually, manufacturers put cornstarch in confectioner's sugar to avoid formation of clumps. For those people who have corn allergies, eating foods with confectioner's sugar may bring adverse effects to their health.

You will feel less pain.

- Inflammation is usually caused by excessive sugar intake. When your body is suffering from an inflammation, you will feel pain in several body parts. Having inflammation throughout your body will affect the immune system negatively. It nourishes yeast and promotes the proliferation of bacteria. If you consume less sugar, your body will be at ease and feel better.

Discover something you don't know yet.

- You may not believe that there are many delectable foods without sugar. There are a lot of sugar substitutes that you can use to add sweetness to your favorite dishes. Using sugar substitutes will not cause negative effects to your immune system.

These benefits are enough to give you a strong will power for eliminating sugar from your diet.

J.C. Collins

CHAPTER 4- NOW! IS THE TIME TO START

By now you are aware that excess sugar in the body is detrimental to one's health. It can lead to obesity, teeth cavities and health diseases. Mostly, sugar-loaded foods do not have the essential nutrients that the body needs. Therefore, eating foods enriched with sugar is not beneficial for your health.

Many people think that having a sugar-free diet is only about getting rid of sweets, but it is not as simple as that. The sugar - free diet also involves removing carbohydrates from your diet. Carbohydrates must also be eliminated because it will be converted into sugar after digestion. It will be difficult for anyone to avoid sugar, but it will be conducive if you know what foods to eat.

The Guide to Losing Weight on a Sugar-Free Diet

1- *The first thing you must do is to avoid all sugar-loaded foods.*

These include all desserts and pastries containing refined

sugar. Cookies, cakes, ice cream, cereals, candies, chocolates, brownies, pies, and sodas should be removed in your daily menu. If you find it difficult to resist your cravings, get a diabetic recipe book and look for sugar-free recipes for desserts. However, you must know that even though these recipes are sugar-free, they may still be high in calories.

2- *Carbs- The Good and the Bad*

Determine which carbohydrates are bad for you. Rice, white bread, corn, pasta, and potatoes contain large amounts of carbohydrates. It will be difficult to avoid corn since most processed foods contain cornstarch. Drinking beer should also be avoided. If you still want to eat these foods, eat them in moderation. It is ideal to eat whole grains on this diet.

3- *Indulge on staple foods of sugar-free diet.*

These include poultry, fruits, fish, vegetables, lean meats, beef and other sources of protein. You can also consume dairy products. When you eat foods enriched with fiber, the production of hunger hormones decreases.

4- *Control your serving size per meal.*

Even if you eat sugar-free foods, you must still eat foods in moderation. You can download an application that can compute how much food you must eat. It will tell you the preferable serving size for different kinds of food. It is advisable to measure your food intake to monitor your weight.

5- *You must keep a diabetic recipe book at home.*

Although you are not suffering from diabetes, this recipe

book will provide you with delicious yet easy-to-make recipes that are sugar-free.

6- Consult Your Doctor

Before adapting sugar-free diet, you must consult your dietitian first. Bear in mind that this diet is not applicable for everyone. For instance, people who exercise regularly will need a lot of carbohydrates to support the daily activities of their body.

7- Sugar substitutes are made either naturally or synthetically. Natural sugar substitutes like agave nectar and honey are good for your health. Be careful not to consume synthetic sugar substitutes like aspartame. Procuring aspartame may lead to nausea, diarrhea and headache.

To completely guide you on your new diet, you must also know the specific foods you are allowed to eat.

J.C. Collins

CHAPTER 5 – FOODS TO EAT AND NOT TO EAT

Based on Los Angeles Times' research, the average sugar intake of a single American is 22 teaspoons per day. The recommended daily sugar consumption is lower than this amount. This situation is quite alarming since many people are now suffering from sugar addiction. To have a successful diet, you must know what foods you must eat.

Foods to Eat

Instead of eating processed foods, you must consume whole foods to achieve your desired weight. Ensuring that you are eating fewer calories can maximize your weight loss. Here are some of the foods you are allowed to eat:

Non-starchy vegetables

Even if you are allowed to eat vegetables on this diet, you still need to assess whether they are starchy or not. Non-starchy vegetables contain more nutrients and fewer calories. If you eat these foods, you are less likely to be hungry.

- Spinach
  leafy greens
  cucumbers
  cauliflowers
  brussels sprout
  kale
  onions
  mushrooms
  bell peppers
  broccoli and asparagus

Although your diet still requires starchy vegetables, you must ensure that you will only consume them in small portions. Starchy vegetables include potatoes, sweet potatoes, and squashes.

Plain dairy products

Plain dairy products consist of zero sugar and are usually high in calcium, protein and good carbohydrates. Cheese, yogurt and milk are good examples of these products.

Fruits with low sugar

All fruits contain sugar, but they differ in amounts. You must consume low-sugar fruits, as they can provide your body with fiber, vitamins, antioxidants and minerals. Low-sugar fruits include berries, apples and mandarins.

Foods rich in protein

Foods rich in protein can make you full longer than eating foods rich in sugar. By eating these foods, you can overcome your sugar cravings. These include:

- poultry
  meat
  sausage
  plain yogurt
  peanut butter
  tofu
  fish
  eggs
  hard cheese
  cottage cheese
  smoked salmon
  and nuts

Healthy fats

Healthy fats aid in the assimilation of antioxidants that are fat-soluble. Fat-soluble antioxidants are usually found in vegetables and fruits. If the body absorbs these substances, you will less likely to feel hungry. Foods that contain healthy fats include:

- Avocado
  olive oil
  balsamic vinegar
  nuts
  peanut butter
  and vinaigrette

Other options

You are also allowed to consume unsweetened fruit juices. You can have gelatin and unflavored jelly for desserts. You can drink milk, hot chocolate, unsweetened tea, and milk, but it is better to drink more water.

Foods Not to Eat

Any diet will only be effective once you follow the rules. You must know the restricted foods, so that you won't accidentally eat them. Here are some of the foods you are not allowed to eat:

Sugar

Sugar-loaded foods include-

- sugar cane
  beet sugar
  chocolates
  corn syrup
  glucose
  ice cream
  jams
  maple syrup
  sucrose
  table sugar
  cakes
  candies
  brownies
  cookies
  granola bars
  honey
  jellies
  molasses
  coffees
  and cereals

Flour-based foods

You should avoid eating flour-based foods since it can make you gain weight. These include:

- bagel
  cookie

corn cereal
croissant
donut
breadcrumbs
pasta
pretzel
rice flour noodles
sandwich roll
tortillas
wheat bread
cake
cereal
corn flour
biscuits
muffins
lasagna
pizza
rice flour
white bread
and white rice

According to dietitians, the main disadvantage of this diet is the challenge one faces upon eliminating all sugar-based products from his diet. Almost all of the foods consist of at least a single kind of sugar. This is why it is difficult to stick on a complete sugar-free diet. To have an effective diet, one must exert more time and effort in reading product labels to check the ingredients.

J.C. Collins

CHAPTER 6 – HELPFUL TIPS ON HOW TO LOSE WEIGHT EFFECTIVELY

Different hormones and neurochemicals may cause extreme sugar cravings. When the production of hormones and neurochemicals drops, the body will require you to replenish the lost supplies by craving for more sugar. The levels of these substances are constantly changing. Thus, the intensity of your sugar cravings varies from time to time.

Serotonin

- The body requires the production of serotonin when you are stressed. Serotonin is a hormone commonly situated in blood platelets, pineal gland, and intestinal track. This hormone reduces reckless behaviors like pain perception, appetite and sexual needs. When the supply of serotonin is low, you are being more aggressive. Symptoms include less impulse management, insomnia and irritability.

- If you acquire more carbohydrates, there will be more insulin in your blood. Insulin is responsible for eliminating amino acids and sugar from the bloodstream. As a result, tryptophan will be left in the blood. Tryptophan is a hormone that can produce serotonin. If amino acids are absent, then it will be easier for tryptophan to produce serotonin. Therefore, there is a greater tendency to crave for sugar when you are stressed. If you don't want to crave for more sugar, keep yourself away from stress.

Endorphin

- When you are stressed, your body will also need some endorphins to be relaxed. Endorphin is a sleep-inducing hormone. The body needs sugar in order to produce enough endorphins. There are some activities that can also trigger the production of endorphins, like sex and exercise. Therefore, you can do some exercise when you are stressed to prevent yourself from overindulging in sweets.

Neurochemicals

- Neuropeptide Y, abbreviated as NPY, is a neurochemical responsible for ensuring that the body has an adequate supply of carbohydrates. If your blood sugar level is low, NPY will be released, causing you to eat more carbohydrates.

- Galatin is another neurochemical that makes you relax when you're stressed. This is often released when your stored fats are not enough to supply your body with energy.

- Even if these hormones and neurochemicals increase your sugar cravings, you can still resist this by doing alternative ways to reduce stress.

Resisting Your Sugar Cravings

Here are some of the helpful tips you may follow to resist your sugar cravings.

Examine the foods you eat.

- Not reading the nutritional facts on the food label is what most people used to do when buying goods. It is very important to know the ingredients of the food you eat. This is to make sure that the foods you will eat are sugar-free. Find "Added Sugar" on product labels. This indicates any ingredient that has been added for adding a taste of sweetness to the product. Added sugar may be in the form of molasses, corn syrup, honey, maltodextrin, syrup, Xylitol, raw sugar, brown sugar, invert sugar, natural sweeteners, dextrin, invert, mannitol, and turbinado sugar. Other forms of sugar usually end with "-ose".

- Remember that the ingredients are arranged in a descending order depending on their quantities. Therefore, the first ingredient that you will see on the list is the main ingredient of the product. If sugar is written on top of the list, then it is not a good option to buy that product.

Your food intake should be comprised of more protein.

- Protein can provide your body with more fuel than the carbohydrates. Many people are confused when they feel hungry. When the body needs protein, your mind is being confused between eating sweets and protein. Since most people like

27

to eat sweets, they would prefer to indulge in sugar instead of protein.

- You must eat foods rich in protein for breakfast. If you have more energy at the start of the day, you will not feel hungry easily. Here are several food options for protein consumption.

- Seafood has less fat content. However, salmon is an exception to that, but it can provide the body with omega-3 fatty acids and healthy oils.

- Dairy products can provide the body with vitamin D and calcium.

- Lean beef is high in protein, iron, vitamin B12 and zinc.

- White meat such as turkey and chicken is high in lean protein. The skin of the meat should be removed since it contains a lot of saturated fats.

- Eggs are a good source of protein. The yolk contains more protein than the egg white.

- Soybeans and peanuts are good options for vegetarians. You can decrease your cholesterol level when you eat soybeans.

Create a meal plan

- It is advisable to eat small amounts of food per meal. In this way, you can maintain your blood sugar level in its normal state and stop regular cravings.

- Eating small portions of food can also prevent indigestion, which is caused by overeating. Many people eat 5 small meals per day. These include a breakfast, lunch, dinner and 2 snacks in between of the major meals. You may set a schedule and create a meal plan, so that you will prevent yourself from craving for other foods.

Fiber is beneficial to your health.

- Fiber reduces the rate of absorbing carbohydrates. Foods rich in fiber are ideal for snacks. These include cereal, oatmeal with fruits, banana, carrots, sweet potato, popcorn with butter, granola bar, whole wheat bread, and sunflower seed.

Remove sweets from your eyesight.

- The best way to avoid sugar is to remove all types of sweets from your eyesight. Clean your pantry and refrigerator. In this way, you will not be stressed in resisting temptations. If there are no sweet foods at home, you don't have any choice aside from eating healthy foods. The activity of cleaning up is already a good exercise for you to be relaxed. Research proved that exercise can decrease your anxiety attacks and provide you more time to focus.

- Shopping for foods should not be done if you are hungry because you may be drawn by your sugar cravings once you see different sugar-loaded foods. You can eat a snack ahead of time, so that you will not be hungry when you are at the grocery.

Eat healthy fruits and vegetables.

- Your digestive system can digest fruits faster than the artificial sweeteners used for making processed foods and sweets. Fruits contain the essential nutrients needed by the body and they are minerals, enzymes, fiber and vitamins.

- Fruits can also reduce the rate of absorbing ingested sugar with the use of its fiber. You can try eating banana, cantaloupe, pear, apple, blueberry, orange, tangerine, and strawberry.

- Rather than eating a slice of cake, you may get some raw vegetables and eat them. Otherwise, you can create a delicious smoothie by blending vegetables, yogurt and ice together. You may also freeze some fruits and squash them.

Only consume healthy fats.

- Many people avoid eating fats, but there are some fats that you should eat. Monounsaturated and polyunsaturated fats are healthy for your body. These fats are commonly found in olive oils, peanuts, hazelnuts, eggs, almonds, and coconut butter. Remember that foods labeled as "low-fat" are mostly rich in sugar. Therefore, you must avoid buying and eating low-fat products.

Resist temptations by doing exercise regularly.

- If you exercise regularly, you will have a consistent supply of serotonin, endorphins, and energy. Serotonin and endorphin have the ability to remove your stress and make you relax. When you crave for sugar, you can distract yourself by being active. You can go out for a walk, run or jog. If you love dancing, you can perform belly dancing or hip hop. Yoga can also calm your mind and relax your body. Trying martial arts would be a great experience. You can also try Tai Chi and Kempo.

Drink more water.

- Since the hunger and thirst signals are released by hypothalamus, your body may be confused between the two. You may think that you are hungry, but the truth is you are only thirsty. Your body may be dehydrated and wants you to drink more water. If you're thirsty, drink a glass of water instead of drinking soda.

- The advisable amount of water you must drink in a day is 8 glasses. You can also drink some herbal teas to hydrate your body.

Dark chocolate is a better option than white and milk chocolates.

- You can still eat some chocolates even if you are on a diet. Dark chocolates have high levels of antioxidants, which can avert type-2 diabetes, tooth decay and heart disease. Chocolates can stimulate phenylethylamine. This is a hormone responsible for happy feelings. As the quantity of phenylethylamine increases, your serotonin level also increases. Thus, your sugar cravings will be lessened if you eat small portions of dark chocolate. You can buy dark chocolates that have 70 percent cocoa. There are more antioxidants in chocolates with more cocoa. Eat chocolates sparingly to avoid disrupting your diet.

Boost vitamin B levels in your body.

- The body's adrenal gland has an important function in regulating stress reactions. If stress persists, there is a greater tendency that you will crave for more sweets. To keep your adrenal gland healthy, you must increase the level of vitamin B in your body. You can take vitamin B-complex supplements regularly. Otherwise, you may eat foods high in vitamin B such as eggs, meats, leafy greens, nuts, milk, fish, whole grains, and fruits.

Artificial sweeteners should be avoided.

- Artificial sweeteners do not help your body to curb sugar cravings. Even though they do not stimulate sugar cravings, these additives may cause several health diseases such as cancers and brain damage. Commonly used artificial sweeteners are saccharin, neotame, aspartame, and sucralose. Even if diet sodas and slimming foods are sugar-free, they are rich in artificial sweeteners that may negatively affect your body.

Consume foods rich in chromium daily.

- Chromium can also help you lose weight. It is a substance that will help your body sustain and balance the blood sugar level. You can take chromium supplements daily. The preferable amount is 600-1000 mcg per day. This dosage must be divided into 3 takes. However, this is not applicable for people who are suffering from diabetes. Foods rich in chromium include barley, green beans, romaine lettuce, broccoli, black pepper, oats, and tomatoes.

Use cinnamon for flavoring your dishes.

- Rather than adding in sugar to your tea, cereal, and oatmeal, you can use cinnamon to add flavor to these dishes.

- Cinnamon can help in regulating your blood sugar level. Consume ¼ teaspoon of cinnamon daily to decrease insulin resistance and regulate low-density lipoprotein cholesterol.

Give your body some time to rest

- Enough sleep may help you lose weight. When you don't have enough sleep, the rate of metabolism may slow down. Metabolism is the process of converting raw materials into energy. Thus, a slower rate of metabolism results to more fats being stocked in the body.

- Sometimes, you cannot avoid sleeping late at night because of work, assignments and other stuff. People tend to grab energy drinks, coffee or chocolates to boost their energy level. However, this solution is only short-lived. After the effects of energy-boosting drinks, your body will require more sugar and thus, you may gain more weight. Taking a nap is the best choice to regain your energy.

- It is important to give your body some time to relax. You can meditate, take a bath, listen to music or close your eyes to relax your mind and body. An adult must have at least 6-8 hours of sleep to keep the body healthy and to decrease the amount of stress. If you experience insomnia, you may drink a glass of warm milk before sleeping.

At the start, you may feel irritated since sugar-free diet has a lot of food restrictions. With enough motivation and effort, you can surpass these challenges to lose weight consistently.

A FINAL WORD

Anyone wishing to maintain a healthy weight and good health should seriously consider cutting sugar from their diet permanently. Experts say sugar addiction takes three days to break. During the detoxification period, health experts recommend treatments such as colonic irrigation as it helps to clean the body and flush out the cells adding hydration. Just think of the long term savings on health bills and looking forward to a slimmer body.

The next step is to apply the things you have learned in real life. You must follow the rules strictly to achieve the best results.

Please Leave a Review

Finally, if you enjoyed this book, please take the time to share your thoughts and post a review on Amazon. It would be greatly appreciated.

That review and feedback will help me improve the content in my books – and make each and every one more relevant and helpful to you.

Thank you again and good luck!

J.C. Collins